Paleo Diet For Beginners

Lose Weight, Feel Great & Start Thriving Living the Paleo Lifestyle

Including 40 Delicious Recipes

Sara Elliott Price

Published in The USA by:

Success Life Publishing

125 Thomas Burke Dr.

Hillsborough, NC 27278

Copyright © 2015 by Sara Elliott Price

ISBN-10: 1511850663

Disclaimer

Every effort has been made to accurately represent this book and its potential. Results vary with every individual, and your results may or may not be different from those depicted. No promises, guarantees or warranties, whether stated or implied, have been made that you will produce any specific result from this book. Your efforts are individual and unique, and may vary from those shown. Your success depends on your efforts, background and motivation.

The material in this publication is provided for educational and informational purposes only and is not intended as medical advice. The information contained in this book should not be used to diagnose or treat any illness, metabolic disorder, disease or health problem. Always consult your physician or health care provider before beginning any nutrition or exercise program. Use of the programs, advice, and information contained in this book is at the sole choice and risk of the reader.

Table of Contents

Introduction

Walking into a modern supermarket can be overwhelming. The sheer volume of choices eclipses common sense, making it difficult to select anything from the sea of shiny packages. If you are trying to keep yourself and your family healthy, the prospects are daunting. Every day, an onslaught of print, television and internet advertising trumpets the latest fat and sugar-laden snack food, and these foods are often advertised side-by-side with the newest diet plan.

How to make sense of it? An increasing number of people are overweight or obese, including children. Pick up any package and read the ingredient list, but get a degree in chemistry first if you want to learn about what you are eating. The prevailing ideas about which foods are healthy to eat, and which are not, frequently change. One day all fat is bad; the next some fats are good. Monday it is fine to eat some carbohydrates; Tuesday all carbohydrates are evil. It's enough to drive anyone crazy.

The array of choices is even more mind-boggling, if you take a look at the limited choices available to our caveman ancestors. Cavemen ate what they could find. They did not have refined sugar, cultivated grains or trans-fatty acids. Based on what we know about nutrition, we can also surmise that there was less obesity than there is today.

The Paleo Diet is part of a movement to simplify things. Complications may seem like a necessary part of modern life, but it is surprisingly easy to simplify things if you try. Processed foods are ubiquitous and inexpensive, but it does not mean that they are healthy. They may look more natural on a busy night as you make dinner for your family, but are they saving you time and money, when you factor in the costs of obesity, illness and lethargy?

The Paleo Diet can help you to narrow down the choices to those that are healthiest for you, and shorten your shopping time by eliminating time spent picking through processed foods.

Eating healthy and losing weight would be reason enough to try the Paleo Diet, but there are additional health benefits that go far beyond weight loss. The combinations of ingredients found in many popular foods in your supermarket may cause or contribute to chronic diseases, including diabetes, coronary artery disease, and autoimmune disorders. What if, in addition to losing weight, you could eliminate or reduce the symptoms of these illnesses, or even make it less likely that you or a loved one gets sick in the first place? The Paleo Diet can help with all of these things.

Chapter 1:
You Are What You Eat

In the United States today, over sixty percent of adults are overweight. As recently as the 1950's, that number was half of what it is in 2014. Why is this? Sometimes, the response to that question is long and complicated, but this section will discuss some reasons for the dramatic increase in obesity, and what you can do to counteract them.

Perhaps the most obvious difference between the 1950's and 2014 is that so many jobs are sedentary. The opportunities of you spending most of your time sitting at your computer are a very high possibility. You might get up to get coffee or to chat with a colleague, but most of the time you're sitting, not standing. You may go to the gym or go for a walk, but when you're at home, you are probably sitting too –in front of the television, or in front of the computer. Time goes by fast, so it wasn't that long ago that most jobs –and most lives –were highly physical. Your ancestors may have been farmers, or tradesmen. They spent their days in hard physical labor, not sitting at a desk.

Another change is that many families now have two working adults. That translates to less family time, less cooking time, and a higher likelihood that families are eating take-out or natural processed foods. Who has time to cook when it is faster to call and order a pizza, or pop something into the microwave? Many people consume their meals on the run, or in front of the television.

In this same period, governmental nutritional guidelines have changed over and over. Following food pyramid recommendations, and balancing those guidelines against the hundreds of diet plans available, can seem impossible. The government tells you to eat a high percentage of carbohydrates, including grains. Other diets tell you to avoid carbohydrates and eat large amounts of animal protein. One food says fat is healthy; another says you should avoid it. Certainly there were diet plans available sixty years ago, but the sheer number of them today presents an unprecedented challenge. How can you know what to eat? The obesity epidemic is in the news, but even with good-faith efforts to turn the tide, the problem is getting worse.

The number one problem is obesity, but it is not the only problem that is caused by the way we eat. Diseases like diabetes, cancer, Alzheimer's disease, Parkinson's disease, infertility and others are rampant, and the way we eat may be contributing to the proliferations of those ailments. More and more people have been diabetes since it is on the rise.

In other words, our nutrition and health are getting away from us. Where does the Paleo Diet enter the picture?

Cave Men didn't eat Twinkies

Our caveman ancestors ate very differently than we do. They did not have supermarkets or fancy packaging. They lived on the land, hunting and gathering what they could eat and then move on. They ate lean wild meats, vegetables and fruits. They did not cultivate food; they found it and ate what they found. Finding food was, in and of itself, a challenge. Lacking methods to preserve or transport what they found, their diets were of necessity both local and seasonal. They consumed what they found when they found it, and with minimal processing. Cooking is a process, so they cooked animal protein and prepared the vegetables and fruits they gathered for consumption.

There were no pesticides available. If a drought or insect attacked a particular type of plant, there was no way to counteract that. In order to survive, they had to find something else to eat. They could not irrigate the tree to alleviate the drought, or genetically alter the tree to ensure it would bear large colorful fruits.

If a caveman consumed and enjoyed an apple and wanted another, but apples were out of season, he had to wait until they were back in season and hope he found one. He could not step into the market and buy an apple from the other side of the planet. He had to make do with what he found when he found it.

Because our ancestors did not cultivate food or process it, their diets were vastly different from the way we eat today. The modern diet includes highly refined carbohydrates like sugar, flour and high-fructose corn syrup. Things like corn and wheat are staples of our diet, not just as ingredients in the food you eat, but in the food your food eats. Cattle, chickens, even farmed fish, eat corn to make them fat and tasty. Left to their own devices, though, animals would eat grass, chickens would eat insects, and fish would eat other fish.

A caveman would not know what to do with a box of pasta. He might try to eat it, but it's unlikely he would recognize it as food. The packaging alone might spook him! He would not recognize many of our modern foods: packaged snacks like Twinkies or cookies; frozen foods and luncheon meats would be foreign to him. Food manufacturers today process their products beyond recognition.

Evolution and your digestive system

Health issues may arise so you finally start asking yourself: why should I eat like a caveman? You may be thinking that human beings have evolved as quickly as our food has, so why should you modify the way you eat?

The answer to that is simple. On a basic genetic level, we are practically identical to our caveman ancestors. The difference between Neanderthal DNA and your DNA is only 0.12%. What that means is that, from a genetic standpoint, we are all more than 99% Neanderthal.

Neanderthals lived in Eurasia as much as 600,000 years ago and died out as recently as 14,000 years ago. More modern humans took their place, and our DNA has not changed much since then.

Humans first cultivated food about 10,000 years ago. The first processed foods became widely available a hundred years ago. Humans have been in an unprecedented period of growth and progress for the past one hundred years, but have our genes kept up with our growth?

Some experts believe they have not. Human beings are extraordinarily adaptive, but technology is moving faster than we are in some ways. We enjoy more comforts and options than ever before. The question is, is it good for us to be changing so quickly? Is there a benefit to slowing things down, putting on the brakes, reconnecting with ourselves on a genetic, ancestral level?

Proponents of the Paleo Diet believe there is a benefit to that approach. Many of the foods you eat today may be contributing to weight gain, obesity, diabetes and other diseases. Milk and other dairy products are one example of foods that may be doing more harm to our health than we realize. Our caveman ancestors did not drink milk beyond early childhood, and even then they drank only the milk their mothers produced because they did not keep or travel with livestock. 65% of the human population has some degree of lactose intolerance, or an inability to properly digest the proteins found in milk. These numbers are higher in parts of Asia.

Evolutionarily speaking, the foods we eat have outstripped our ability to understand them correctly. This is true not only of dairy; it's true of cultivated grains like corn and wheat; vegetable oils; refined sugars; and so many others. Eating these foods can cause diseases like diabetes, cancer and Celiac disease.

The Paleo Diet will help you to eliminate the foods that may cause digestive problems, and eat those foods that promote good digestion and overall health and well-being. It is a way of streamlining both your diet and your life, consuming whole foods that are easy to digest and prepare and eliminating those that contribute to weight gain, disease and chronic pain.

Chapter 2:
Connecting With Your Inner
Hunter/Gatherer

What can I eat?

As you begin your day, you're probably thinking, "What can I eat? "If cookies, potato chips, and frozen dinners are out, then what foods left for you to eat?

Like the Paleo Diet itself, the answer is simple. You can eat a wide variety of vegetables and fruits, and lean animal protein. If it is in the package (unless it's a package of fresh or frozen vegetable) chances are it is a highly-processed food and therefore not a part of the Paleo Diet. It is also important to note that hunter/gatherers ate food that they found above the ground, so while an occasional sweet potato is excellent, for the most part stick to what lives and grows in plain sight. Tree nuts are good; legumes and ground nuts like peanuts are not.

While in general you can eat as many vegetables as you need, there are guidelines to help you figure out how much of your diet should come from protein. A typical Paleo plate should be 2/3 vegetables with a palm-sized portion of protein and small amounts of fruit and healthy fat. If you are trying to lose weight, you will need to be cautious about eating too much fruit as the sugar content is high and can contribute to weight gain.

While cavemen ate only what is seasonal and local, the Paleo Diet is not quite as restrictive. You may eat any of the fruits and vegetables you see at your local supermarket, as long as you are eating them as they are, and not as part of a processed food. In other words, fresh broccoli is a yes, broccoli pizza is a no.

The animal protein part of the diet is a little trickier, primarily because it's not as simple as just buying some chicken. Huge agricultural companies gather livestock in confined spaces and force feed them corn and other foods which may or may not be in their natural diet. Eating the Paleo way means that you will need to be mindful not only of what you eat, but what of what the animals you consume ate as well. You may want to believe that's impossible and shouldn't matter at all, but it is not as complicated as it sounds. First, let's talk about how governmental nutritional guidelines are different from those on the Paleo Diet.

Contrasting the Paleo Diet with nutritional guidelines

You have probably seen a food pyramid at some point in your life. A food pyramid is typically a visual representation of the diet the government recommends. Recent versions place grains and grain products at the bottom of the food pyramid, recommending ten to twelve servings per day.

Cavemen did not eat much grain. While we cannot know for sure what cavemen ate, we do know that human beings did not cultivate their food until 10,000 years ago. Prior to that, early humans ate what they found, and then moved on. Plants, vegetables and fruits were their dietary staples, not grains.

The next tier of the government food pyramid reserved for fruits and vegetables, followed by dairy and animal protein and ending with fats and sweets at the top. On the Paleo Diet, you will eat vegetables, fruits and lean animal protein, and healthy fats like olive oil and coconut oil mostly.

How to hunt and gather in a modern supermarket?

Most modern supermarkets have similar layouts. The design requires shoppers to navigate a maze of aisles where shelves overflow with a mind-boggling array of processed foods to get from one end of the store, where the fruits and vegetables be, to the other end of the store, where the meats and fish. Many people choose processed foods over fresh ones on occasion, and some of us do it every day.

It's understandable, but in the end, it is also unhealthy. How can you avoid those traps? The answer is surprisingly easy: shop the perimeter.

The next time you walk into your local grocery store, stop for a minute and take a careful look at the different sections. You must take your time and look, you will see that the fresher, less processed foods like fruits, vegetables, eggs and meats are in the front of the store; while the highly processed foods in cans, boxes and freezers are in the middle. If you are shopping and your child pleads for a sweet snack, he or she probably saw it in the middle aisles of the store. You may need to avoid those aisles filled with temptation and go down the aisles with Paleo-friendly items that will help you adapt to your new lifestyle.

Many grocery stores have the produce section at the front of the store, right where customers enter. That's awesome news for you, because you can start your shopping in the healthiest way possible. Here you have the advantage over your caveman ancestors because the vegetables and fruits are all together in this section. In the caveman era, their food supply didn't consist of a wide variety of fruits and vegetables available to them a year-round like we have it now.

Stock up on green leafy vegetables like spinach and kale and fiber-rich cruciferous vegetables like broccoli and cauliflower. Take note of which vegetables your children enjoy, and buy those regularly, and find recipes (there are some at the end of this book) that will induce them to try some new things.

The produce section is not without its pitfalls. You will need to be cautious with high-sugar fruits like bananas and pineapple; and with starchy vegetables like potatoes. These are still healthier than processed foods, but they are also high in sugar. If weight loss is your goal, eating too much sugar may make it more difficult to lose the extra weight you are carrying. Organic foods are more expensive than their non-organic counterparts, but if you want to avoid pesticides and chemicals, buy organic.

A special note about corn: In the Paleo Diet, corn in considered a grain, not a vegetable. Corn is one of the most widely-used ingredients in processed foods, and it is very difficult to avoid if you are not careful. Not only is it an ingredient, but it is also a component of things like high-fructose corn syrup and corn sugar. In addition, big livestock companies and food manufacturers feed their cows, chickens and pigs a corn diet, meaning that corn may be an ingredient in your hamburger!

Frequently you can find dairy products at the back of the grocery store. Milk, cheese and other dairy products are not part of the Paleo Diet. Nearly 65% of the human population has some degree of lactose intolerance, and cavemen did not milk cows. However, they would probably have eaten eggs. The best choice for the Paleo Diet is eggs because of the high levels of Omega-3 fatty acids, preferably eggs that are from cage-free chickens. Caged chickens often eat a diet of corn, which is not something a chicken would eat if left to its resources. The right eggs are a healthy and satisfying part of the Paleo Diet.

A great part of the Paleo Diet may surprise you. Even though cavemen didn't keep cows, butter from grass-fed cows is part of the Paleo Diet. If you are sensitive to lactose, try using ghee (clarified butter) instead of butter. You will need to avoid vegetable oils high in polyunsaturated fat and Omega-6 fatty acids. Some good choices include olive oil, as it's almost completely mono-unsaturated fat and coconut oil, as well as animal fat. Apply the same guidelines to animal fat that you would to animal protein.

Finally, don't skip the meat and seafood sections. Here again, you will need to exercise some caution regarding corn. Stick to grass-fed beef, free range chicken and wild-caught fish, and avoid corn-fed beef, caged chicken meat and farm-raised fish.

Chapter 3:
Did Cavemen Have Diabetes?

Now you understand the basics of the Paleo Diet, but you may still have questions about what it can do for you. You have probably guessed that the Paleo Diet can help you lose weight. The diet is naturally low in carbohydrates. You would need to start by eating a lot of broccoli in order to match the carbohydrates in a bowl of pasta. The Paleo Diet allows you to fill up on healthy foods, making it easier to slim down and get your body in shape, but weight loss is only the beginning of what the Paleo Diet can do for you.

The rate of diabetes among the general population has nearly doubled in the past sixty years or so. Eating processed foods with a high glycemic index (a rating of food on a scale from 1 to 100, measuring the effect that a given food has on your glucose, or blood sugar, levels) forces the body to produce insulin. A study has shown that eating too much of these foods may cause you to develop diabetes since your family have a history of it. It makes the Paleo Diet a good choice for people with diabetes or high blood sugar, because the majority of foods that make up the Paleo Diet have a low glycemic index. If you have high blood sugar, diabetes or a familial tendency toward diabetes, you will need to limit your intake of fruit to 2-

3 pieces a day, and choose fruits with a lower glycemic index. For example, oranges, apples and kiwis have a lower glycemic index than bananas and grapes. Charts listing the glycemic index of favorite foods are widely available on the internet.

It is crucial that you reduce your risk of heart disease by following the Paleo Diet. While there are various causes of heart disease, including obesity, lack of exercise and diet, some research suggests that the primary factor in heart disease is inflammation. Because the Paleo Diet includes foods rich in Omega-3 fatty acids, is contained in a number of foods that are anti-inflammatory, which means that eating this way can help reduce your risk of heart disease. Examples of Omega-3 rich foods are wild salmon, Omega-3 enriched eggs and walnuts.

Another benefit of eating a diet rich in Omega-3 fatty acids is better brain function. You probably don't think of your food as affecting your brain, but it does. Many Americans who consume a typical diet may not be getting sufficient Omega-3 fatty acids, which include docosahexaenoic acid (DHA). Doctors use DHA to treat premature babies because it stimulates mental development. DHA is an ingredient in baby formula for the same reason. Furthermore, DHA is a treatment for diabetes, dementia, and coronary artery disease, and it can improve vision, prevent macular degeneration and even help prevent or minimize depression.

Eating the Paleo way can also help improve your digestive health. Evolutionarily speaking, you are not that different from your caveman ancestor, but chances are your current diet contains at least a few things that you are not able to digest properly. Foods high in fat and sugar can overload your body. It can only process so much of what you take in, and the rest gets stored as fat. The combination of highly processed foods with a stressful lifestyle may also cause something called "leaky gut syndrome. "It sounds horrible, and it is. What it means is that the food can leak out of your intestinal tract and end up where it doesn't belong.

Some diets consisting mostly of fruits and vegetables are also a nutritionally complete diet. While daily vitamins pills are a convenience, nutritionists believe that it is best to get vitamins from food. Processed foods may sometimes have added vitamins and minerals –check out the side of a cereal box –but they're added artificially during the manufacturing process.

Eating a wide variety of vegetables (a good guideline is choosing vegetables in different colors, since the color is often a sign of the vitamins a vegetable contains) will certainly ensure that you are receiving enough of the vitamins you need to be healthy. It can, in turn, lead to more energy because foods with a low glycemic index take longer to digest. That means these foods supply you with long-lasting energy and leave you feeling full, too.

No Pain, No Grain: Autoimmune disorders and the Paleo Diet

What is an autoimmune disease? Diseases that impair your body's immune responses, causing it to attack the proteins within your body as if they were foreign cells. Recent studies suggest that all autoimmune diseases are linked to inflammation of the digestive system. Some conditions that fall into this category are Irritable Bowel, Celiac Disease, Crohn's Disease, and Rheumatoid Arthritis. In Rheumatoid Arthritis, for example, your body attacks the connective tissue in your joints, causing pain and limiting movement.

How does the Paleo Diet help with these disorders? You already know that the Omega-3 fatty acids in the diet help reduce inflammation. Diet plays a significant part in the development of Rheumatoid Arthritis and the severity of its symptoms. Because the Paleo Diet eliminates many of the foods that cause inflammation, it may help those with Rheumatoid Arthritis. Some experts suggest that people with this disease should also eliminate eggs, nuts, and certain fruits and vegetables, eggplant and spicy peppers.

Approximately 1% of the general population has Celiac disease, in which consumption of foods containing gluten (such as wheat) causes inflammation of the small intestine. Celiac Disease is hereditary, but if you have it, you can help manage the symptoms by following the Paleo Diet. The Paleo Diet is naturally low in gluten because it does not include grains such as wheat and barley. Some studies show that people with Refractive Celiac Disease (an unusually severe form of the disease that can cause cancer) whose symptoms did not improve on a gluten-free diet went into complete remission when following a Paleo Diet.

In short, the Paleo Diet goes far beyond weight loss. Eating Paleo is a lifestyle that can improve your overall health.

Chapter 4:
Losing Weight the Paleo Way

Donuts don't grow on trees

Eating processed foods is one of the biggest hindrances to sustained weight loss. Why? Why do eating packaged and processed foods cause us to put on weight and keep it on? One theory is that many processed foods include both sugar and fat, a combination that never exists in nature. Animal protein has fat but very little sugar. Most fruits and vegetables are very healthy, and the few that are high in fat (avocados, for example,) are very low in sugar. In other words, donuts don't grow on trees.

It's not just the combination of sugar and fat that makes processed food dangerous. Look at the ingredient list on any highly processed food. Chances are that in addition to sugar (including number one diet offender high-fructose corn syrup) you will also find a list of unpronounceable chemicals. Some are flavor enhancers; some are stabilizers, and some are preservatives. No matter what the reason for their inclusion, though, they are not natural and may have effects far beyond those intended by the manufacturer.

The truth is that most processed foods send your digestive system and metabolism into a tailspin. Your body cannot process the chemicals and highly refined carbohydrates, and when it comes to carbohydrates, what you do not consume gets turned into fat and stored in your body. You already know that eating these foods can lead to leaky gut syndrome and autoimmune deficiencies, but they may be making you fat as well.

Eliminating these foods is the first step toward losing weight the Paleo way. Once you stop eating them, you can replace them with healthier, Paleo choices like lean protein, and large amounts of vegetables, as well as healthy fats and eggs. A Paleo omelet in the morning can keep you full for hours, increasing your energy and productivity and helping you lose weight.

Eat as much as you want and still lose weight

If you've ever been on a diet –any diet –you know how difficult it can be to lose weight. Proponents of each diet claim impressive results, complete with before and after photographs and enthusiastic testimonials. Why is the Paleo Diet different? For starters, there are no calorie restrictions on the Paleo Diet. The reason that very low calorie diets do not work in the long term is because they put your body into starvation mode. When that happens, your metabolism slows to make the calories you do take in last longer. That makes it very difficult to sustain weight loss.

How can the Paleo Diet eliminate calorie restrictions? It's simple, really. You must adhere to the guidelines of the Paleo Diet; you can eat your fill of healthy foods because they are lower in carbohydrates, higher in Omega-3 fatty acids, and more satisfying. You must consume ten cups of broccoli to match the calories in one fast food cheeseburger. Many vegetables are high in dietary fiber, which contributes to a feeling of fullness.

The same is true of the animal proteins that are part of the Paleo Diet. Protein keeps you feeling full and satisfied longer than carbohydrates do.

To lose weight on the Paleo Diet, you will still need to monitor your intake of certain foods. Fruit is an excellent example. Sugar in any form can make it difficult to lose weight, so limit your fruit intake to two or three pieces a day, and avoid high-sugar options like bananas and pineapple. Good alternatives are grapefruit, apples and pears. You should also avoid highly processed vegetable oils, like corn oil and canola oil, and use healthier options such as coconut oil, palm oil or olive oil.

Because vegetables, fruits and lean protein are the focus, the Paleo Diet is an excellent choice for people who struggle with carbohydrate cravings and high blood sugar. The elimination of things like refined carbohydrates, sugars and caffeine may be painful for the first three days your body is trying to get use to your new way of eating.

Eating out on the Paleo Diet

Restaurant dining while on any diet can be a challenge, and the Paleo Diet is no different. Restaurant food is often high in fat, including vegetable oils and salt. Some may wonder if they can eat out and still adhere to the Paleo Diet.

The answer is yes. You just make some special requests when your order is taken to avoid consuming non-Paleo foods. The first thing you may want to do is to ask questions. Don't be afraid to ask if fish is wild or farmed, for example, or if beef is corn or grass-fed. You need to ask your waiter or waitress before they take your order, various questions about all the ingredients put in each dish, and how the chef prepared the food: what type of fats the chef is using, for example. Your server will know or will be able to get answers to your questions quickly since most restaurants are more than happy to help with special requests.

Once you have determined which things on the menu are Paleo-friendly, the next step is to check out the menu as a shopping list rather than a fixed set of options. If wild salmon is on the menu, you do not need to order it with the mashed potatoes that accompany it. You can ask for a side of broccoli, or a salad, or anything else that is on the menu. You can specify what kind of oil you want your food cooked in (coconut or palm oil may be a stretch, but most restaurants will have olive oil) and how much salt is on your food. Ordering this way may take some practice, but it will soon become second nature.

Chapter 5:
Cooking Like a Caveman In a Modern Kitchen

Now that you understand the Paleo Diet and how it works, it's time to put what you've learned to practice in your kitchen. You've got a refrigerator full of fresh vegetables and fruits, lean protein and Omega-3 rich eggs. You've gathered the right kinds of oil, as well as some nuts. You're ready to cook like a caveman would, if a caveman had a modern kitchen to work.

Breakfast

Paleo Omelet

Ingredients:

- 2 cage-free eggs (or Omega-3 enriched eggs)
- ¼c. chopped onion
- 8 oz. cubed chicken
- ½c. mushrooms, sliced
- 1 clove crushed garlic
- ½tsp. chopped sage
- 1 Tbsp. coconut oil, olive oil or ghee

Method on the next page.

Method:

1. Heat the oil in a frying pan. After you heat the pan, add the onion and garlic.

2. While the onions are simmering, crack the eggs into a bowl and whisk them to blend.

3. When the onion is translucent pour the eggs into the pan and tilt it, so they cover the bottom of the pan evenly. As the edges of the eggs set, use a spatula to push the eggs toward the middle of the pan so the uncooked eggs will spread out and cook.

4. After 2-3 minutes, put the mushrooms, chicken and herbs on top of the eggs.

5. Next, let it continue to cook until the eggs fully set (5 minutes or so) then use a spatula to turn one side of the omelet and fold it toward the center.

6. Repeat on the other side. Serve with hot sauce to taste.

This recipe is very easy to adapt. Substitute 8 oz. cubed ham for the chicken, use spinach or tomatoes in place of the mushrooms, or basil in place of the sage.

√+

Paleo Blueberry Muffins

Ingredients:

- 2 1/2 c. almond flour
- 1 Tbsp. coconut flour
- 1/4 tsp. salt
- 1/2 tsp. baking soda
- 1 Tbsp. vanilla
- 1/4 c. coconut oil
- 1/4 c. maple syrup
- 1/4 c. coconut milk
- 2 eggs
- 1 c. fresh or frozen blueberries
- 2-3 Tbsp. cinnamon

Method:

1. Preheat oven to 350. Line a 12 count muffin tin and lightly oil.
2. In a mixing bowl combine flours, salt, and baking soda—stir to combine.
3. Pour in coconut oil, eggs, maple syrup, coconut milk and vanilla. Mix until well blended.
4. Fold in blueberries and cinnamon. Pour evenly into muffin liners.
5. Bake 22-25 minutes.

27

Almond Butter Pancakes

Ingredients:

- 1/2 c. almond butter
- 1/2 c. unsweetened applesauce
- 2 eggs
- 1/2 tsp. baking soda
- 1/2 tsp. cinnamon
- 1/2 tsp. vanilla

Method:

1. Preheat oven to 350 and line baking sheets with parchment paper (a must to prevent sticking).
2. In medium bowl combine all ingredients and mix until well blended and batter consistency.
3. Scoop batter onto lined baking sheets using 1/4 c. measuring cup. I usually end up with around 6 pancakes. You may need two baking sheets to prevent touching.
4. Bake 10-12 minutes until fluffy and golden. Enjoy with maple syrup.

Paleo Egg Muffins

Ingredients:

- 12 cage-free eggs
- ¼c. cooked chopped spinach
- ¼c. chopped tomatoes
- 1 Tbsp. chopped basil
- Salt and pepper to taste
- Coconut oil, olive oil or ghee
- Preheat the oven to 350 degrees

Method:

1. You start by cracking several eggs, place them in a bowl and whisk.
2. Then season the eggs with the salt and pepper to give it flavor.
3. Add the vegetables and herbs and mix.
4. Use your preferred oil to grease a muffin tin (12 muffins) and then divide the egg mixture evenly into the tins. Place the tin in the oven and bake for 20 to 25 minutes or until the eggs are fully set.
5. Wait until the eggs cool for a 4 to 5 minutes, and then you can remove them from the pan and enjoy. You can place the eggs in the refrigerator for a several days, so

they are an excellent option for hectic mornings because they are portable.

Like the omelet recipe, these are readily adaptable. Different variations might include bok choy with ginger and a little coconut aminos, zucchini and mushrooms, or bacon and chives. If you want to make several different sets at once, simply divide the egg mixture into separate bowls.

Winter Fruit Compote

A winter fruit compote uses reconstituted dried fruit.

Ingredients:

- ½ cup pitted prunes
- ½ cup dried apples
- ½ cup dried cherries
- ½ teaspoon cinnamon
- ¼ teaspoon powdered ginger
- Pinch of salt

Method:

1. Place the fruit, spices and salt in a saucepan and cover with water.
2. Bring to a boil over medium heat. Reduce heat and simmer for 5 minutes.
3. Turn off the heat and allow the fruit to absorb the liquid for 2 hours, or until fruit is plump.

Spiced Coconut Cereal

Ingredients:

- 1 tablespoon ground cinnamon
- 1 teaspoon ground nutmeg
- 1 tablespoon plus 1 teaspoon organic vanilla extract
- 1/2 teaspoon stevia powder
- 1/2 cup water
- 1 cup unsweetened coconut flakes

Method:

1. Preheat the oven to 300 degrees F. Line 3 cookie sheets with parchment paper.
2. In a large bowl, add all ingredients except coconut flakes and beat till well combined.
3. Transfer the coconut flakes in prepared cookie sheets evenly.
4. Bake for about 15 minutes. Remove the cookie sheets from oven and stir the flakes.
5. Bake for 5 to 10 minutes further.
6. Remove from oven and let the flakes cool completely.
7. Transfer this cereal into an airtight container and preserve in refrigerator for 1-2 weeks.
8. You can enjoy this cereal with any non-dairy milk and fruit's topping.

Chia Seeds Breakfast Pudding

A totally satisfying breakfast recipe without any fuss... This enchanting mix of blueberries, banana, dates and chia seeds make a gorgeous and delicious breakfast treat.

Ingredients:

- 2/3 cup unsweetened almond milk
- 2 cups frozen blueberries
- 1/2 of a frozen banana, peeled and sliced
- 5 large soft dates, pitted and chopped
- 1/2 cup chia seeds

Method:

1. In a food processor, add all ingredients except chia seeds and pulse till smooth.
2. Transfer the mixture into a bowl.
3. Add chia seeds and stir to combine well.
4. Refrigerate for 30 minutes, stirring after every 5 minutes.

Simple Bread

√+

Ingredients:

- 1/3 cup almond flour
- 1/2 teaspoon baking powder
- Salt, to taste
- 2 1/2 tablespoons coconut oil
- 1 organic egg

Method:

1. Grease a microwave safe mug.
2. In a bowl, mix together flour, baking powder and salt.
3. In another small bowl, add oil and egg and beat well.
4. Mix egg mixture into flour mixture.
5. Transfer the mixture into prepared mug.
6. Microwave on high for 1 minute 30 seconds.
7. Let it cool for about 5 minutes.
8. Carefully remove from mug and cut into 2-4 equal sized slices.
9. You can serve this bread with the topping of maple syrup.

Chocolate Waffles

A deliciously fun breakfast recipe for chocolate lovers.

Ingredients:

For Waffles:

- 1 cup blanched almond flour
- 1/3 cup coconut flour
- 1/3 cup cacao powder
- 1/2 teaspoon baking soda
- Salt, to taste
- 4 organic eggs
- 1 cup applesauce
- 1/2 teaspoon organic vanilla extract
- 1/3 cup 70% dark chocolate chips

For Sauce:

- 1/3 cup 70% dark chocolate chips
- 2 tablespoons coconut oil

Method:

1. Preheat the waffle iron on high.
2. In a large bowl, mix together flours, cacao powder, baking soda and salt.

3. In another bowl, add eggs, applesauce and vanilla and beat till well combined.

4. Add egg mixture in the bowl with flour mixture

5. and mix till well combined.

6. Gently, fold in chocolate chips.

7. Pour about 3/4 cup of mixture in waffle iron. Cook for about 4-5 minutes.

8. Repeat with the remaining mixture.

9. Meanwhile for sauce in a small pan, add chocolate chips and coconut oil on low heat.

10. Cook, stirring continuously till the chocolate chips melt completely,

11. Serve the waffles with the topping of chocolate sauce.

Paleo Crepes

Ingredients:

- 3 tablespoons coconut flour, sifted
- Salt, to taste
- 6 large organic eggs
- 1 cup unsweetened almond milk
- 2 tablespoons coconut oil, melted
- 2 tablespoons coconut oil, for cooking

Method:

1. In a bowl, mix together flour and salt.
2. In another bowl, add eggs, milk and 2 tablespoons of melted oil and beat till well combined.
3. Add egg mixture in the bowl with flour mixture and mix till well combined.
4. Heat 1 tablespoon of oil in a crepe pan or a nonstick skillet on medium-high heat.
5. Place 1/4 cup of mixture in pan and immediately tilt the pan so the mixture spreads thinly in the whole pan.
6. Cook for about 1 minute. Carefully flip the side and cook for about 15 seconds.

<u>Lunch</u>

Taco Lettuce Wraps

Ingredients:

- 1 lb. ground turkey
- 1 medium onion, diced
- 1 can chiles in adobo sauce
- 1 c. diced tomatoes
- ¼ c. sliced scallions
- 1 avocado, cubed
- 12 lettuce leaves, rinsed and patted dry
- 1 Tbsp. olive oil or ghee

Method:

1. Heat up the oil in a skillet. Add the onion and cook on medium heat until translucent.
2. Add the turkey and cook it thoroughly.
3. While the turkey is cooking puree the chiles in adobo to make a quick sauce. When the turkey is nearly finished cooking, add the adobo sauce and continue to cook until heated through.
4. Lay out the lettuce and spoon the turkey mixture into the leaves. Garnish each one with tomatoes, scallions and avocado.

Simple Salmon

Ingredients:

- 32 oz. filet of salmon
- 1 lemon, sliced thin
- 1 Tbsp. capers
- Salt and pepper
- 1 Tbsp. fresh thyme
- Olive oil, for drizzling

Method:

1. Line a baking sheet with parchment paper and place salmon, skin side down. Season with salt and pepper.
2. Place capers on the salmon and top with lemon and thyme.
3. Put the baking sheet in a cold oven, then turn oven up to 400 degrees F. Bake about 25 minutes.

Goes well with a nice green salad with a vinaigrette dressing.

Paleo Chopped Salad

Ingredients:

- 2 c. dark leafy greens, roughly chopped
- 2 tomatoes, chopped
- 1 cucumber, chopped
- 1 avocado, diced
- 1 c. chicken, diced
- Lemon vinaigrette (recipe follows)

Method:

1. Carefully, put all the ingredients in a large mixing bowl and stir them all together.

Dress with lemon vinaigrette. Find this dressing on the next page.

Lemon Vinaigrette

Ingredients:

- 3 Tbsp. fresh lemon juice
- ¾c. olive oil
- 1 clove garlic, minced
- Salt and pepper to taste

Method:

Traditional vinaigrette recipes call for drizzling the oil into the lemon juice or vinegar while whisking or blending in a food processor. An easier method is simply to put the ingredients into a jar then screw the lid on tight and shake until fully emulsified.

When it comes to making this recipe, you can substitute lime juice if you prefer, or apple cider vinegar and experiment with different herbs and spices. This simple lemon vinaigrette is good on almost any salad, and you can use it as a sauce for chicken or shrimp, too.

Chicken Tortilla Soup

Ingredients:

- 2 large skinless chicken breasts, cut into 1/2 inch strips
- 1 28 oz. can diced tomatoes
- 32 oz. organic chicken broth
- 1 sweet onion, diced
- 2 jalapeños, de-seeded and diced
- 2 c. shredded carrots
- 2 c. chopped celery
- 1 bunch cilantro chopped
- 4 cloves garlic, minced
- 2 Tbsp. tomato paste
- 1 tsp. chili powder
- 1 tsp. cumin
- salt and pepper to taste
- olive oil
- 1-2 c. water

Method:

1. Add all ingredients to a slow cooker, adding enough water to fill to top and cook on low for 2-3 hours.
2. Before serving you can shred the chicken easily for a more authentic dish.
3. Top with avocado slices and fresh cilantro.

Lemony Egg Soup

Ingredients:

- 1 tablespoon olive oil
- 1 tablespoon garlic, minced
- 6 cups chicken broth, divided
- 2 organic eggs
- 1 tablespoon arrowroot powder
- 1/3 cup fresh lemon juice
- Freshly ground white pepper, to taste
- Fresh chopped parsley, for garnishing

Method:

1. In a large soup pan, heat oil on medium-high heat.
2. Add garlic and sauté for about 1 minute.
3. Add 5 1/2 cups of broth and bring to a boil on high heat.
4. Reduce the heat to medium. Simmer for about 5 minutes.
5. Meanwhile in a bowl, add eggs, arrowroot powder, lemon juice, white pepper and remaining broth and beat till well combined.
6. Slowly, add egg mixture in the pan, stirring continuously.
7. Simmer, stirring continuously for about 5-6 minutes.
8. Serve hot with the garnishing of parsley.

Green Gazpacho

A creamy gazpacho great for a light lunch. The addition of avocado makes this cold soup deliciously creamy without adding any dairy product.

Ingredients:

- 1 medium cucumber, peeled, seeded and chopped
- 1 small avocado, peeled, pitted and chopped
- 1 tablespoon onion, chopped 1 garlic clove, chopped
- 1 tablespoon fresh lemon juice
- 1 tablespoon olive oil
- 1 tablespoon apple cider vinegar
- 1/4 teaspoon red chili powder
- Salt, to taste
- 1 cup water
- Smoked paprika, for garnishing

Method:

1. In a blender, add all ingredients except paprika and pulse till smooth.
2. Serve with the garnishing of paprika.

Tuna Salad Filled Avocados

Tuna salad filled avocados make a great, quick and easy lunch. This dish gets its creaminess from avocados and packs a punch of onion and fresh lemon juice.

Ingredients:

- 1 large avocado, halved and scooped out the flesh from middle
- 1 tablespoon onion, chopped finely
- 2 tablespoons fresh lemon juice
- 5-ounced cooked tuna
- Salt and freshly ground black pepper, to taste

Method:

1. In a bowl, add scooped out avocado flesh, onion, and lemon juice and mash till well combined.
2. Add tuna, salt and black pepper and stir to combine.
3. Divide the tuna mixture in both avocado halves evenly.
4. Serve immediately.

Prawns & Veggie Curry

A mild and tasty prawn and veggie curry for the whole family. This tasty curry is a great choice for you to introduce your children to spicy foods for the first time.

Ingredients:

- 2 teaspoons coconut oil
- 1/2 medium white onion, sliced
- 2 medium green bell peppers, seeded and sliced
- 3 medium carrots, peeled and sliced thinly
- 3 garlic cloves, chopped finely
- 1 tablespoon fresh ginger, chopped finely
- 2 1/2 teaspoons curry powder
- 1/2 pounds prawns, peeled
- 1/2 tablespoons red boat fish sauce
- 1 cup coconut milk
- 2 tablespoons water
- 2 tablespoons fresh lime juice
- Salt and freshly ground black pepper, to taste
- 2 tablespoons fresh cilantro leaves, chopped

Method:

1. In a large skillet, heat oil on medium-high heat.
2. Add onion and sauté for about 1-2 minutes.

3. Add bell peppers and carrot and sauté for about 3-4 minutes.
4. Add garlic, ginger and curry powder and sauté for about 1 minute.
5. Add prawns and fish sauce sauté for about 1 minute.
6. Add coconut milk and water and stir to combine.
7. Cook, stirring for about 3-4 minutes.
8. Stir in lime juice and remove from heat (season with salt and black pepper if required).
9. Serve hot with the garnishing of cilantro.

Baked Mixed Veggie Meatballs

These healthy baked meatballs are packed with the flavors of ground beef and a variety of fresh vegetables and herbs.

Ingredients:

- 1/2 cup carrot, peeled and grated
- 1/2 cup zucchini, grated
- 1/2 cup yellow squash, grated
- Salt, to taste
- 1 pound grass-fed ground beef
- 1 organic egg, beaten
- 1/3 of a small onion, chopped finely
- 1 garlic clove, minced
- 2 tablespoons mixed fresh herbs (parsley, basil, cilantro - chopped finely)

Method:

1. Preheat the oven to 400 degrees F. Line a large baking sheet with parchment paper.
2. Set a large colander in the sink. Add carrot, zucchini and yellow squash and sprinkle with 2 pinches of salt.
3. Keep it for at least 10 minutes. Transfer the veggies over a paper towel and squeeze out all the moisture of veggies.

4. In a large mixing bowl add squeezed vegetables, beef, egg, onion, garlic, herbs and desired amount of salt and mix till well combined.

5. Shape the mixture in desired and equal sized balls. Arrange the meatballs into prepared baking sheet in a single layer.

6. Bake for about 25-30 minutes or till done completely.

7. Enjoy these balls with fresh veggie salad.

Dinner

Spaghetti Squash and Meatballs

Ingredients:

- 1 large spaghetti squash
- 1 lb. grass-fed ground beef
- 1 large cage-free egg
- 1 16 oz. can tomatoes
- 1 large onion, diced small
- 3 cloves garlic, minced
- 2 Tbsp. olive oil
- dried basil
- dried oregano
- dried thyme
- salt& pepper
- fresh basil

Method:

1. Preheat the oven to 450 degrees.
2. Start by slicing the spaghetti squash in half and remove the seeds with a spoon.
3. Take your baking pan or cookie sheet and line it with foil, and then you brush the inside of the spaghetti squash using olive oil, and seasoned with little salt and pepper to give it a great taste.

4. You have to cook the squash with the cut side facing down in the pan for 40 minutes. Let cool.

5. Fix the meatballs, mix the ground beef with the egg and dried spices, salt and pepper to taste.

6. Roll the mixture to form small meatballs.

7. Get a large pot, heat up the oil while cooking the onions and garlic on medium until the onions are translucent.

8. You can brown the meatballs beforehand, or simply cook them together with the sauce.

9. Add the tomatoes, dried spices and salt and pepper to the pot, and drop the meatballs into the sauce.

10. Cook on medium-low heat until the meatballs are cooked thoroughly.

11. When the spaghetti squash is cool, use a fork to remove the squash out of the skin. If you scrape it lengthwise, the squash will resemble thin spaghetti.

12. Pile the "noodles" into bowls and top with the meatballs and sauce.

13. Garnish with fresh basil ribbons and serve.

Serves 4

Paleo Stir Fry

Ingredients:

- 1 ½lbs. grass-fed beef, cubed
- 1 medium onion, sliced
- 1 c. broccoli florets
- 1 c. mushrooms, sliced
- ½c. carrots, sliced
- 2 scallions, sliced
- 1 Tbsp. fresh ginger, grated
- 2 Tbsp. fresh cilantro, chopped
- Low-sodium soy sauce
- 2 Tbsp. coconut oil
- Salt and pepper

Method:

1. You must heat half of the oil in a large non-stick skillet, season the beef with salt and pepper, as it cooks in a skillet, and then put it in a bowl.
2. Put the rest of the oil left over in the pan along with the onions until they are translucent.
3. Add the remaining vegetables, but make sure you put the vegetables that will take the longest to cook first on the stove (carrots first, then broccoli).

4. After the vegetables thoroughly cook, add the browned meat along with the scallions, ginger, cilantro and soy sauce.

5. You can enjoy eating this as is, or put it into lettuce leaves and serve it as a wrap.

Serves 4

Texas Style Chili

Ingredients:

- 4 lbs. grass fed stew meat cut into 1.5 in. cubes
- 2 lbs. pork shoulder cut into 1.5 in. cubes
- 2.5 lbs. tomatoes roughly chopped
- 2 onions roughly chopped
- 1 lb. of various chile peppers (pick based on how hot you like your chili) roughly chopped
- 6 cloves of garlic, chopped
- 3 Tbsp. smoked paprika
- 3 Tbsp. cocoa powder
- 2 Tbsp. ground cumin
- 1 tsp. salt
- 1 tsp. black pepper

Method:

1. Season meat with salt and pepper and rest at room temperature for 1 hour.
2. Sear meat over medium-high heat until all sides of all meat are browned.
3. In a large bowl, toss tomatoes, garlic, paprika, cocoa powder, cumin, salt and pepper.

4. Add to the slow cooker bottom to top the following. Add onions to the bottom, then chilies, the meat, and finally add the tomato/ spice mixture.

5. Turn your slow cooker on low and cook for 10 hours. To thicken the sauce, remove the lid for the last hour of cooking. Taste and season as needed.

6. Serve with your favorite toppings, such as green onion, fresh tomatoes, or paleo crackers.

Zucchini Noodles/Sweet Potato Noodles

A simple side dish that can be done two ways, with zucchini or sweet potato. If you have elevated blood sugar or diabetes, the zucchini is a better option.

Ingredients:

- 2 large or three medium zucchini

OR

- 2 large sweet potatoes

- 1 clove garlic, minced
- 1 Tbsp. olive oil or ghee
- 1 tsp. chopped fresh thyme
- Salt and pepper

Method:

1. Using a vegetable peeler scrape large ribbons from the side of the zucchini or sweet potatoes (peel the sweet potatoes first.) Scraping lengthwise will give you the longest noodles. Scrape as many noodles as you can, and then save the centers for another recipe.
2. Once you have your noodles ready bring a large pot of water to a boil. Salt the water and blanch the noodles

(the sweet potato will take a bit longer than the zucchini, plan on one minute for the zucchini and 2-3 minutes for the sweet potato.)

3. Remove the noodles and put them into a quick ice water bath, and then pat them dry.
4. Heat up the olive oil or ghee in a skillet, add the garlic, and then stir in the noodles. These won't take very long to cook, so watch them make sure they don't burn.
5. Toss and serve.

These are an excellent accompaniment to grilled salmon, steak or chicken.

Grilled Whole Chicken

Ingredients:

- 1/4 cup olive oil
- 2 tablespoons fresh lemon juice
- 1 teaspoon dried oregano, crushed
- 1 teaspoon onion powder
- 1 teaspoon garlic powder
- 2 teaspoons paprika
- 2 teaspoons fresh lemon zest, grated finely
- Salt and freshly ground black pepper, to taste
- 1 (4-pound) grass-fed whole chicken

Method:

1. Preheat the grill to medium heat. Grease the grill grate.
2. In a bowl, add all ingredients except chicken and mix till well combined. Keep aside.
3. Place chicken on a cutting board, breast side down.
4. With a sharp knife cut along both sides of the back bone and then remove the back bone.
5. Flip the breast side up and open it like a book. With the palm of your hands press breast firmly to flatten.
6. Coat the whole chicken with oil mixture generously.
7. Grill for 16-20 minutes, flipping once halfway.

Chicken with Bell Pepper and Cashew

An authentic chicken dish with a sweet and nutty flavor and a touch of spice.

Ingredients:

For Chicken:

- 2 pounds grass-fed skinless, boneless chicken thighs, cut into bite-sized pieces
- 2 tablespoons arrowroot powder
- Salt and freshly ground black pepper, to taste
- 2 tablespoons coconut oil
- 2 red bell peppers, seeded and chopped
- 1 1/3 cups raw cashews
- 1 large scallion bunch, chopped

For Sauce:

- 1 tablespoon fresh ginger, grated finely
- 3 garlic cloves, minced
- 1/4 cup coconut vinegar
- 1/3 cup coconut aminos
- 3 tablespoons coconut palm sugar
- 2 tablespoons homemade tomato paste
- 1/2 teaspoon red pepper flakes, crushed

Method:

1. In a large bowl add chicken, arrowroot powder, salt and black pepper and toss to coat well. Keep aside.
2. In a large skillet, heat oil on medium-high heat.
3. Add bell peppers and sauté for about 2-3 minutes. Transfer the bell pepper in a bowl.
4. In the same skillet, add chicken mixture and stir fry for about 5-8 minutes.
5. Meanwhile in a bowl, add all sauce ingredients and beat till well combined.
6. Ad sauce, stirring continuously. Stir in cashews and bell peppers. Bring to a gentle simmer.
7. Reduce the heat to medium-low. Simmer for about 3-5 minutes or till desired thickness.
8. Stir in scallion and serve.

Grilled Sirloin Steak with Herbs

A classic recipe with the perfect combination of steak and marinade. This nice marinade of fresh herbs with vinegar, garlic and seasoning adds a refreshing flavor to the steak.

Ingredients:

- 1 cup extra-virgin olive oil
- 3 tablespoons red wine vinegar
- 2 shallots, minced
- 3 garlic cloves, minced
- 3 tablespoons fresh basil, minced
- 2 tablespoons fresh thyme, minced
- 2 tablespoons fresh rosemary, minced
- 2 tablespoons fresh parsley, minced
- 2 teaspoons dried oregano, crushed
- Salt and freshly ground black pepper, to taste
- 2 (15-ounce) grass-fed beef sirloin steaks

Method:

1. Preheat the grill to high heat. Grease the grill grate.
2. In a bowl, add all ingredients except steaks and mix till well combined.
3. Transfer half of herb mixture in a large bowl.
4. Add steaks and coat with herb mixture generously. Keep aside for about 20 minutes.

61

5. Grill for about 5-7 minutes on both sides.
6. Rub the remaining herb mixture on both sides of steaks evenly.
7. With a sharp knife, cut the steaks in desired slices and serve.

Ground Beef with Greens

Ingredients:

- 1 tablespoon olive oil
- 1/2 of white onion, chopped
- 2 garlic cloves, minced
- 1 jalapeno pepper, chopped
- 1 pound grass-fed ground beef
- 1 teaspoon ground coriander
- 1 teaspoon ground cumin
- 1/2 teaspoon ground fennel seeds
- 1/2 teaspoon ground ginger
- 1/2 teaspoon ground cinnamon
- 1/2 teaspoon ground turmeric
- Salt and freshly ground black pepper, to taste
- 8 cherry tomatoes, quartered
- 1 bunch fresh collard greens, trimmed and chopped
- 1 teaspoon fresh lemon juice

Method:

1. In a large skillet heat oil on medium heat.
2. Add onion and sauté for about 4-5 minutes.
3. Add garlic and jalapeno and sauté for about 1 minute.
4. Add beef and spices and cook, stirring occasionally for about 6-8 minutes.

5. Add tomatoes and greens and cook for about 4 minutes.
6. Stir in lemon juice, desired salt and black pepper and remove from heat.

Salmon with Parsnip Pasta

Ingredients:

- 1 (4-ounce) skinless salmon fillet
- 1 tablespoon fresh lemon juice
- 1/2 tablespoon olive oil
- Pinch of dried oregano, crushed
- Salt and freshly ground black pepper, to taste

For Parsnip:

- 2 teaspoons extra-virgin olive oil
- 1 leek, chopped
- 1 garlic clove, minced
- Pinch of red pepper flakes, crushed
- 2 medium parsnips, peeled and spiralized with blade
- 2 tablespoons homemade vegetable broth
- 2 teaspoons fresh parsley, chopped
- 1 lemon wedge

Method:

1. Preheat the oven to 425 degrees F. Line a small baking sheet with parchment paper.
2. Place the salmon fillet onto prepared baking sheet.
3. Drizzle with lemon juice and oil evenly and sprinkle with oregano, salt and black pepper.

4. Bake for about 20-25 minutes. Remove from oven and with a fork flake the fillet.
5. Meanwhile for parsnips use a large skillet, heat oil on medium heat.
6. Add leeks, garlic and red pepper flakes and saute for about 1-2 minutes.
7. Stir in parsnips and broth and cook covered for about 5-7 minutes.
8. Stir in flaked fillet and cook for about 1 minute.
9. Serve with the garnishing of parsley and lemon wedge.

Curried Prawn with Veggies

A warming curry recipe that will be a great addition to your dinner menu list.

Ingredients:

- 2 teaspoons coconut oil
- 1/2 medium white onion, chopped
- 1 tablespoon fresh ginger, minced
- 2 medium green bell peppers, seeded and sliced thinly
- 3 medium carrots, peeled and sliced thinly
- 1/2 pounds prawns, peeled and deveined
- 3 garlic cloves, minced
- 2 1/2 teaspoons curry powder
- 1/2 tablespoons red boat fish sauce
- 1 cup coconut milk
- 2 tablespoons water
- 2 tablespoons fresh lime juice
- Fresh cilantro, for garnishing

Method:

1. In a large skillet, heat oil on medium-high heat. Add onion and sauté for about 1-2 minutes. Add ginger and sauté for about 30 seconds.
2. Add bell peppers and carrots and cook for about 4-5 minutes.

3. Add prawns, garlic, curry powder and fish sauce and stir fry for about 30 seconds.
4. Add coconut milk and water and cook, stirring for about 3-4 minutes.
5. Stir in lime juice and remove from heat.
6. Serve hot with the garnishing of lime juice.

Snacks

Roasted Cauliflower

Ingredients:

- 8 c. cauliflower florets
- ¼c. olive oil
- 4 cloves garlic, minced
- 2 tsp. fresh herbs, chopped (thyme, rosemary, or parsley)
- Dash of cayenne pepper
- Salt and pepper to taste

Method:

1. Preheat oven to 450 degrees.
2. Layer the cauliflower into a baking dish and mix it with the other ingredients.
3. Bake until the cauliflower is golden brown – about 20 minutes.

This is delicious just as it is, as a snack or even a side dish. If you want a different texture (and a great substitute for mashed potatoes) try pureeing this in your food processor.

Note: This method is also an excellent way to cook Brussels sprouts. The only difference is the cooking time. Roast at 450 for 45 minutes.

Apple Slices Dipped in Dark Chocolate

Ingredients:

- 1/4 c. lemon juice or apple cider vinegar
- 2 medium apples, type of your choosing
- 3 oz. high quality dark chocolate, chopped
- 2 Tbsp. walnuts, chopped

Method:

1. Add lemon juice or vinegar to a medium bowl, then fill with water until 2/3 full. Set aside.
2. Core and quarter the apples into slices. Thickness will depend on how you prefer them to be sliced. Place slices into lemon juice and water mixture to soak—this prevents browning.
3. Now, melt the chocolate in a microwave safe container in 30 second intervals to ensure it doesn't burn. Stir every 30 seconds until melted. Finely chop walnuts and place in a small dish.
4. Line baking tray with wax paper.
5. Drain apple wedges and pat dry with paper towel. Dip each apple wedge into the chocolate and place on wax paper.
6. Sprinkle on walnuts.
7. Repeat for each apple slice.

8. Transfer tray to fridge so chocolate can harden, and then serve.

Kale Chips

Ingredients:

- 1 bunch kale
- 1 Tbsp. olive oil
- Sea salt

Method:

1. Preheat oven to 350 degrees.
2. After removing the ribs the kale, cut it into bite-sized pieces.
3. Rinse the pieces and thoroughly dry them in a salad spinner.
4. Toss them with olive oil and salt to taste, and then spread them in a single layer on a cookie sheet.
5. Bake them for 10-15 minutes (you'll have to watch it) until the edges are brown and the chips are crispy.

Baba Ganoush with Crudité

Ingredients:

- 1 large eggplant
- 1 Tbsp. olive oil
- 2 cloves garlic, minced
- 1 Tbsp. flat-leaf parsley, chopped
- Salt and pepper

Method:

- Preheat oven to 450 degrees.
- Slice the eggplant in half, brush it with olive oil and then sprinkle with little salt and pepper.
- Place it in a pan and cook for at least 20 to 25 minutes or until soft.
- Wait until it is cool enough to remove it from the pan and eat.
- Let some of the excess liquid drain from the eggplant (hold it over the sink or a plate to do this) and then scoop the cooked eggplant into a food processor.
- Add the garlic, parsley and additional salt and pepper if desired, and puree until the mixture is smooth.
- Serve with cut fresh vegetables (cauliflower and broccoli florets, celery, carrots, etc.)

Fried Chicken Wings

A mouthwatering recipe of pan fried chicken wings. The spicy and tangy marinade adds a really refreshing sticky, spicy and zingy flavor to chicken wings.

Ingredients:

For Marinade Mixture:

- 1 teaspoon fresh lemon zest, grated finely
- 2 large garlic cloves, minced 2 teaspoons coconut oil, melted
- 1 tablespoon fresh lemon juice
- 1 1/2 tablespoons coconut aminos
- 2 teaspoons tomato paste
- 2/3 teaspoon ground coriander
- 2/3 teaspoon onion powder
- 2/3 teaspoon salt

For Chicken:

- 14 grass-fed chicken wings
- Coconut oil, for cooking

Method:

1. In a large bowl, mix together all marinade ingredients.
2. Add chicken wings and coat with marinade generously.

3. Cover and refrigerate to marinate for at least 1 hour.
4. In a large skillet, heat oil on medium heat.
5. Add chicken wings, skin side up. Cook for about 2 minutes.
6. Then cover the skillet and cook for 4 minutes.
7. Uncover and flip the side.
8. Cook for about 2 minutes.
9. Then again cover the skillet and cook for 4 minutes more.

Crispy Fish Sticks

A really delicious and nutritious snack recipe. These delicious baked fish sticks are moist on the inside and crunchy on the outside.

Ingredients:

- 1 cup arrowroot flour
- 2 large organic egg whites
- 2 1/2 cups pork rinds, crushed
- 2 tablespoons fresh parsley, minced
- 2 1/2 teaspoons fresh lemon rind, grated very finely
- 1/2 teaspoon freshly ground black pepper
- 2 pounds cod fillets, cut into 3/4-inch wide and 3-inch long sticks

Method:

1. Preheat the oven to 425 degrees F. Lightly, grease a large baking dish.
2. In a shallow dish, place arrowroot flour.
3. In second, shallow dish, add egg whites and beat well.
4. In third shallow dish mix together remaining ingredients except fish sticks.
5. Roll the fish sticks in arrowroot flour completely. Then dip in egg whites. Then roll in pork rind mixture completely.

6. Arrange the chicken strips into prepared baking dish in a single layer.

7. Bake for about 8-10 minutes or till done completely.

Sweet Potato Croquettes

These super simple but yummy baked sweet potato croquettes need only 5 ingredients.

Ingredients:

- 3 cups cooked sweet potato, peeled and mashed
- 2 tablespoons grass-fed salted butter
- Pinch of salt
- 2 organic eggs
- 1 cup almond meal

Method:

1. Preheat the oven to 400 degrees F. Line a large baking sheet with parchment paper.
2. In a bowl mix together mashed sweet potato, butter and salt.
3. In a shallow dish crack the eggs and beat well.
4. In another shallow dish place almond meal.
5. With a tablespoon take mixture of sweet potato make balls and flatten them slightly.
6. Dip the croquettes in beaten eggs.
7. Then roll in almond meal completely.
8. Arrange the croquettes onto prepared baking sheet in a single layer.
9. Bake for about 25-30 minutes or till done completely.

Apricots Squares

Ingredients:

- 1 cup raisins
- 1 cup raw almonds, chopped roughly
- 1/2 teaspoon ground cinnamon
- 10 dried apricots, chopped
- 1/2 cup unsweetened coconut, shredded

Method:

1. In a food processor add raisins, almonds and cinnamon and pulse till smooth.
2. Add apricots and pulse a little. Then, add coconut and pulse till well combined.
3. Transfer the mixture between 2 sheets of parchment paper placed onto a cutting board.
4. With your hands, press the mixture to form square shape.
5. Place the wrapped mixture in refrigerator for about 20-30 minutes.
6. Remove from refrigerator. With a sharp knife cut the mixture into 25 equal sized squares.

Blueberry Protein Bites

A sweet and sinfully satisfying snack that is high in protein. These no bake protein bites taste like delicious blueberry muffins.

Ingredients:

- 1 scoop Paleo friendly unsweetened protein powder
- 1/2 cup coconut flour, sifted
- 1-2 tablespoons coconut palm sugar
- 1/4 teaspoon ground cinnamon
- Pinch of sea salt
- 1/4 cup dried blueberries
- 1/2-1 cup almond milk

Method:

1. Line a large cookie sheet with parchment paper. Keep aside.
2. In a large bowl, mix together all ingredients except almond milk.
3. Gradually add desired amount of almond milk and mix till dough is formed.
4. Immediately make desired sized balls from mixture.
5. Arrange the balls onto prepared baking sheet in a single layer.
6. Refrigerate to set for about 30 minutes.

Lemony Cookies

Ingredients:

- 1/4 cup pure maple syrup
- 1 cup cashew butter
- 1 teaspoon fresh lemon zest, grated finely
- 2 tablespoons fresh lemon juice
- Pinch of salt

Method:

1. Preheat the oven to 350 degrees F. Line a large cookie sheet with parchment paper.
2. In a food processor add all ingredients and pulse till smooth.
3. With a tablespoon place the mixture onto prepared cookie sheet in a single layer.

Bake for about 12 minutes or till golden brown.

Kids and the Paleo Diet

If you have children who have been eating a high volume of heavily processed foods, getting them to eat Paleo can be a real challenge. First, try making small changes, and don't introduce too many new things at once.

Kids love to eat peanut butter, but it's not allowed on the Paleo Diet, but you can try giving them almond butter instead. Add skewered vegetables (cherry tomatoes, cucumbers, whatever they like) in their school lunches. After they've adapted to each new thing, present something else. The egg muffins in the Breakfast section are an excellent choice for children and are a natural substitute for high-sugar breakfast cereals.

You can try things like breading chicken with almond or coconut flour and making chicken nuggets. Most ketchup is very high in sugar, so serve them with a simple marinara sauce. For lunches, roll up vegetables in slices of roast beef or turkey (matchsticks of zucchini and carrot work well with this, with some avocado for creaminess) or pack some of the taco lettuce wraps (recipe in the Lunch section) so they can make their tacos at school. The main ingredient here is patience, since many children will be resistant to change.

Conclusion

Now that You've learned a lot about how the Paleo Diet works, are you are ready to get started. Before beginning, you may want to purge your kitchen of foods that are not Paleo friendly. Removing processed foods from your home will make it easier to follow your new diet. It may be very difficult if other people in your house, like your spouse or children, are not following the diet, but try to remove the processed foods that are a temptation to you. Even if other people in your family are not following the Paleo Diet, as you introduce a new way of eating they may decide to join you.

After you've cleared your home of unhealthy processed foods, head to the supermarket to hunt and gather the foods you will need for your new lifestyle. If you remember to shop the perimeter of the store, it will be easier to stick to the foods that are on the Paleo Diet. If you are shopping for others and find that you need things from the center aisles, your new knowledge of the Paleo Diet may also help you to make healthier choices for your family, even if they are not eating the Paleo way. Read the labels, and try for options that do not include unhealthy ingredients and chemicals.

Since you want to lose weight, stay healthy or manage an autoimmune disorder, it's best to speak with your doctor first before starting the Paleo Diet. Your doctor or nutritionist knows how to help you fine-tune the diet so that you are getting the foods that are most important for your particular needs, and avoiding those that are not. With autoimmune diseases, foods that are Paleo friendly, like nuts and certain fruits and vegetables in the nightshade family (tomatoes, eggplant, potatoes and others) may be counterproductive. It is important to do your research before starting to get the best possible results.

When you first start your new Paleo Diet, don't be alarmed because it may take some times for your body to start getting use to your new way of eating. If your diet up until now has included a high amount of sugar and refined carbohydrates, your body will need to accustom itself to the absence of those foods. Be patient with yourself. Make sure to drink plenty of water.

As the Paleo Diet increases in popularity, some food manufacturers are selling things like Paleo bread, or Paleo pie. Keep in mind that just because the package says that the food is Paleo does not mean that it actually is. Hunter-gatherers did not have bread or pie. Eat whole foods as much as possible.

The Paleo Diet can help you lose weight, feel healthier and even alleviate symptoms of autoimmune diseases. Why not try eating like a caveman?

Made in the USA
Middletown, DE
09 March 2016